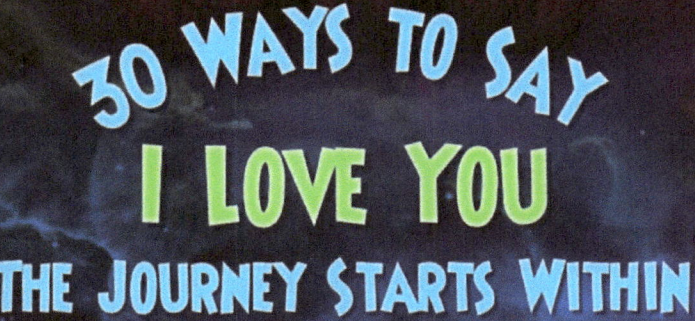

Copyright © 2021 Love_Light91
All Rights Reserved.
HerLife HerWrite Publishing Co. LLC
ISBN: 978-1-7349232-5-4

TO MY PRINCESS JULIANNE,

YOU REKINDLED THE FIRE IN MY SOUL.

TO MY SOUL TRIBE,

THANK YOU FOR YOUR UNCONDITIONAL POSITIVE REGARD, LOVE, AND UNDERSTANDING.

Table of Contents

- ♥ **It all starts with You** — 8
- ♥ **Internal Insights** — 10
- ♥ **Breathe Better** — 12
- ♥ **Hydration Station** — 14
- ♥ **Silent Messages** — 16
- ♥ **Make Time** — 18
- ♥ **Relaxation Station** — 20
- ♥ **Fight for Fuel** — 22
- ♥ **Boundaries Baby** — 24
- ♥ **Mirror Moments** — 26
- ♥ **Fortunate Failures** — 28
- ♥ **Minor Mountains** — 30
- ♥ **Nasty Negatives** — 32
- ♥ **Peace Palace** — 34
- ♥ **Actively Attentive** — 36

Table of Contents

- ♥ Neuro Narrator — 38
- ♥ Balance the Beast — 40
- ♥ Manipulate the Map — 42
- ♥ Childlike Cheerfulness — 44
- ♥ Fiery Faith — 46
- ♥ Recharge Reset — 48
- ♥ Medicinal Meditation — 50
- ♥ Weird and Wonderful — 52
- ♥ Sincerely Selfish — 54
- ♥ Empathetic Exchange — 56
- ♥ Waring with Worries — 58
- ♥ Despite the Difficulties — 60
- ♥ Happy Hiatus — 62
- ♥ Rinse Repeat — 64
- ♥ Healthy Habits — 66

Mission Statement

This is not a traditional book. You can start anywhere, and you may finish where you please.

Change should not be a chore, and neither should this read.

I hope you enjoy each page, and the lesson that it brings.

Body, mind, and soul all on one accord. The journey starts within, and then the limits are no more.

Discloser/Disclaimer

Please consult your physician for personalized medical advice. Always seek the advice of a physician or other qualified healthcare provider with any questions regarding a medical condition. Never disregard or delay seeking professional medical advice or treatment

These statements have not been evaluated by the Food and Drug Administration. This product is not intended to diagnose, treat, cure, or prevent any disease.

It all starts with You

Accountability: an obligation or willingness to accept responsibility or to account for one's actions

Hold yourself accountable by committing to making one positive, maintainable change each day.

My first two commitments were:

1. Today I will commit to waking up 30 minutes early and make time for me.
2. Today I will commit to listening twice as much as I speak.
3. Your turn:
   Today I will commit to…….

Change starts where complaining ends.

Journal Page

Internal Insights

Think of your body as a luxury dream car. Are you going to allow your $20,000 car to go without regularly scheduled maintenance checks?

Then why would you treat your mind, body, and soul any different?

> How I know my check engine light is on:
1. EVERYTHING annoys me!
2. Procrastination replaces motivation.
3. Your turn:

My check engine light is on when:

> Your behaviors tell a story. To fully love you, you have to be willing to relearn yourself.

Journal Page

Breathe Better

Life can hit harder than two fifteen inch subwoofers, knocking the breath smooth out of your mind, body, and soul.

Breathing deeply, mindfully, and purposefully provides you with extra time to reflect on the costs/benefits of reacting or engaging

Here is a guide on one way to breathe better:

1. Close your mouth and inhale quietly through your nose to a silent count of four.
2. Hold your breath for a count of seven
3. Exhale completely through your mouth, making a whoosh sound to a count of eight.
4. Now inhale again and repeat the cycle three more times for a total of four breaths.

Journal Page

Hydration Station

Cracked, peeling, dry, callused feet usually motivate you to apply moisturizer, right?

Having a dry mouth, feeling thirsty, dizzy, tired, inability to focus, and dark yellow urine are sure signs you need to moisturize your insides.

Three steps I take to stay hydrated:

1. Drink one gallon of spring water daily.
2. Add key lime and other seeded fruit to my water for flavor.
3. Eat my water (watermelon, strawberries, peaches, & cucumbers) are my favorites.

What three steps can you take to stay hydrated despite your busy schedule?

Journal Page

Silent Messages

Emotions can be overwhelming, uncomfortable, and sometimes unpredictable. The same goes for lace-front wigs and visiting a new barber.

If you wouldn't allow those things stand in your way of physical transformation, why would you allow these things to stand in the way of you learning and loving more about yourself?

How I check my emotional voicemail:

1. Dig deeper than anger because it is a secondary emotion.
2. Be honest, direct, and intentional about your emotions with yourself and those you choose to interact with.

Journal Page

Make Time

Wake up, prepare the kids, slide a snack, drop them off, clock in, slave, clock out, and finish the list in reverse.

When do you have time for you?! If you wait for the perfect calm moments of life to have time, sadly it will never come.

We have to make time no matter how much or how little as long as it is consistent.

How I make time for me:

1. Wake up 30 minutes early
2. Throughout the day, say positive "I am" statements.
   Examples: I am loved, I am worthy, I am enough.
   How can you make more "me" time?

Journal Page

Relaxation Station

Guilt, anxiety, and shame are the typical feelings associated with relaxation away from adulting.

Pouring from an empty cup only delivers dust and fuss. How much time do you purposefully spend doing absolutely nothing or at least something that helps recharge, refocus, and redirect us to more positive supportive thoughts and behaviors?

Three relaxing activities I enjoy:

1. Reading mystery novels
2. Spending time in nature
3. Making vision board/scrapbook

This week I commit to relaxing by:

1.
2.
3.

Journal Page

Fight for Fuel

The food you eat can impact thoughts, moods, energy levels, sleep patterns, and more.

If you wouldn't put tattoo ink in a laser printer and expect the printer to work, how could you expect to fill up on sugary, fatty, oily, genetically modified and hybrid foods, and still consistently produce organized thoughts, feelings, and actions about yourself? Do not just take my word for it, look it up!

Foods I eat for fuel on the go:

1. Mango fruit
2. Mixed Greens Salad
3. Irish Sea Moss Gel
    . I now challenge you to find three new fuel foods.

Journal Page

Boundaries Baby

Boundaries remind you and inform others of what you will and won't accept, tolerate, or allow.

Setting new boundaries with others as you grow can be hard. Especially, when everyone is used to benefiting from you not having any at all. Do not let this deter you from protecting your growth, peace, and joy.

Boundaries can be applied to every aspect of life (professional, personal, business, individuals, etc.).

How I set boundaries:

1. Say "NO" without explaining why.
2. Be consistent and firm with everyone!
3. Exchange guilt for self-care

Journal Page

Mirror Moments

How many times a day do you find yourself in front of a mirror and avoiding eye contact with yourself for whatever reason?

When you complete a business deal that you whole heartedly intend to carry out, you make eye contact, smile, and shake on it, right?

I took an oath to conduct business with myself in the same manner. Each moment in the mirror, I grow to know and love my business partner more and more.

Mirror Moment Mantras

1. I love you
2. I am healthy, wealthy, and wise.
3. Control is an illusion, go with the flow.

Journal Page

Fortunate Failures

It is through lived experience that you can testify to your growth and progress.

Live life no longer from a sense of deprivation, shame, & guilt due to past, current, and future failures.

Instead, walk in the freedom of accountability. If you can commit to making one small positive change each day, in 30 days you will have 30 new ways to love and appreciate you.

Accountability & Me

1. Journal daily
2. Reframe one "failed" moment of the day to find the silver lining.
3. Give thanks each morning, noon, & night.

Journal Page

Minor Mountains

Our irrational beliefs fuel our irrational responses. Plainly stated, Rule number one to surviving anything….

DON'T PANIC!!!

Let's say you get fired.

The natural response might be, "Oh snap, rent is due, car payment, kid's sports fees, and the tank is on E!".

Minor Mountain response would be, " Well, I was looking for a job when I found this one." Or "It is about time I file for my LLC and EIN number."

What are some minor mountains in your life?

1.

2.

3.

Journal Page

Nasty Negatives

Negativity is contagious. Complainers attract more things to complain about.

I challenge you to THINK before you speak.

T: Is it thoughtful?

H: Is it helpful?

I: Is it inspirational?

N: Is it necessary?

K: Is it kind?

If the answer is no, why speak it into existence?

In everything that you do and say, do so in pure love. Expect nothing in return, and there will be no bridges left to burn.

Journal Page

Peace Palace

Peace is knowing even if the waves flip the boat, I can float.

Keeping the space around you free of clutter is the first step to freeing your mind of the clutter standing in the way of your peace.

Holding on to peace is worth letting go of everything sent to destroy it.

Maintaining My Peace Palace

1. Silence
2. Solutions over Slander
3. Replace fear with preparedness

What about you?

1.

2.

3.

Journal Page

Actively Attentive

We are actively attentive to our phone notifications, our supervisor's requests, and several other demands of life.

Being actively attentive to yourself includes but is not limited to: pausing for a snack, taking a nap, ending a gossip session before it begins, letting people know when you need alone time, etc.,

Learn to listen to the voice in your heart the first time around to avoid an annoying repeated cycle.

What are 2 cues your body uses to alert you and remind you to pay attention?

1.

2.

Journal Page

Neuro Narrator

Awareness is key to success.

Now that you are aware of how to actively listen to yourself, I invite you to start tweaking the narrator voice inside your head.

Replace that dry eyes commercial with a fun, spunky, encouraging, comedic, entertaining voice, and see how much easier it becomes to listen to the cues and navigate the path of learning to love yourself better.

What attributes would make your narrator easier to listen to?

1.

2.

3.

Journal Page

Balance the Beast

Balance is more than just deep breathing while standing on one leg with the other leg extended out in front of your body.

Spiritual, financial, physical, emotional, social, environmental, intellectual, and occupational are all eight dimensions of wellness that require balance for success.

1. Time in nature
2. Budget
3. Exercise
4. Smile
5. Build trust with others
6. Keep respectful company
7. Stimulate your mind
8. Seek inspiration and challenges

Doesn't matter which dimension you choose to start with, all roads lead to loving you

Journal Page

Manipulate the Map

Tired of repeating the same route in life over and over again?

There is always a blessing in the lesson. Once you learn the lesson, get the blessing, and put your life back into gear.

You know what doesn't work for you as evidenced by your current life circumstances.

The decisions you make today direct the steps you take tomorrow.

How I manipulate my map:

1. Stop expecting
2. Observe don't absorb
3. Write down my lesson learned daily

Accountability & Consistency

Journal Page

Childlike Cheerfulness

Children find every reason under the sun to smile.

Ask yourself, will my negative reaction change the outcome? When you discover the answer, remember to smile and find at least one thing to be cheerful about in that very moment.

Observe the impact of this action on your thoughts, feelings, and actions moving forward.

3 Things I am always cheerful about:

1. Being Alive
2. Activity of my limbs & airways
3. To love & be loved

What are you cheerful about today?

1.
2.
3.

Journal Page

Fiery Faith

Faith can be thought of as a chemical in the mind. When unconditional love is mixed with the chemical faith in your mind, it opens a spiritual portal of limitless manifestation.

Know it! Speak it! Manifest it!

Then, take practical steps each day to assist with the manifestation.

Even when things don't add up or make any sense, remember to fuel your focus with fiery faith.

Choose 3 areas of life that would benefit from you having fiery faith:

1.

2.

3.

Journal Page

Recharge Reset

Make it a Routine!

Recharge, rest, and refocus as often as you see fit. At least one day out of the week should be spent encouraging and supporting self.

This does not mean running errands without the kids to the store.

Mindfully schedule activities that allow you to tune in with your higher self. It is time to pour into yourself all of the love, care, and nurturing you provide to others.

My activities:

1. Turn phone on DND
2. Read self-help books
3. Gym time
4. Sleep to sound healing music

What can you do for R&R?

Journal Page

Medicinal Meditation

Have you ever felt like something was a little off, but couldn't quite put your finger on to exactly what was bothering you?

Meditation allows you to quiet the noises around and inside of you. Once everything is quiet, you can begin to hear and understand what you need from you.

Utilize online resources for guided meditations if you are unsure of how to start.

Start small with maybe five minutes of mediation at a time.

Side effects may include but not limited to: Self-love, peace, focus, clarity, motivation, and understanding.

Journal Page

Weird and Wonderful

You are uniquely made after the creator's inspiration.

Weird, wonderful, and waging war against everything sent to convince you of anything less.

If you don't love it, change it. If you can't change it, learn to love it!

Find the shirt that compliments your curves. Hire the life coach for extra support and encouragement. Go talk with the therapist that is bound by law to keep your secrets out the streets.

Do whatever it takes to embrace your weird and wonderful.

What can you embrace today?

1.
2.

Journal Page

Sincerely Selfish

Self-care is mandatory!

This season of your life, I challenge you to be selfish!!!

Selfish with your resources, time, energy, and effort.

Unconditional love does not equal unconditional access!

Exclamation marks because this is one of the foundational pillars to successfully loving you again.

The way you treat you, models how everyone else is going to treat you.

Don't get angry with them, instead, redirect that energy to hold yourself accountable for the example you gave them to follow.

Journal Page

Empathetic Exchange

As an empathetic individual, you may experience the emotions or physical symptoms of those around you.

Try to keep a 3:1 ratio (three positive interactions for every negative interaction you decide to engage with or endure).

Also, as an empath, self-care is very critical to avoid compassion fatigue. As you learn how to observe without absorbing, here are 3 tips to stay afloat.

1. Accept it you are "**different**"!
2. Daily alone time.
3. Learn to listen not labor.
    As empaths, we are naturally "fixers". Today it is time to learn how to redirect that energy back to you boo!

Journal Page

Waring with Worries

The waves of worry hold the potential to drown out the vision that was originally downloaded during your season of fiery faith.

Solutions over sympathy, that is for self as well. IF your thought isn't representative of what you wish to manifest, replace it with your vision, mission, goal, step, encouragement, and support.

Why war with worry when you could manifest with fiery faith and unconditional love?

Stop what you are doing right now, and say these out loud:

1. Control is an illusion.

2. Worry is a waste of good energy.

Journal Page

Despite the Difficulties

Difficulties, challenges, and other barriers to success are going to present themselves on your journey to learning how to unconditionally love yourself.

When difficulties present themselves, pause and ask yourself one simple question: How can I learn and grow from this lesson today?

Be honest with yourself about what you feel and the true internal source and message of that feeling, and allow yourself to exchange offense for accountability.

The dark and difficult times and lessons supply the tools needed to maintain the blessing. Perspective is everything.

Journal Page

Happy Hiatus

Hiatuses, vacations, breaks, time off, etc., will become a regular part of your schedule if you continue to follow this format.

You do not have to earn to deserve rest. It is one of the basic needs for survival.

When you feel guilty about resting your body, mind, heart, and soul, say these affirmations out loud:

1. Rest is required.
2. I am still not stagnant.
3. I must schedule my happy hiatus consistently if I desire to provide myself with unconditional love and positive regard.

Journal Page

Rinse Repeat

Now that you have learned thirty ways to say I love you to your mind, body, heart, and soul, I encourage you to reread as often as necessary.

Take your time, don't apply any pressure to yourself. This should be an organic experience. So, don't feel the need to do them in any set order.

Rinse and repeat until you feel complete.

Then recommend to a friend to help them learn thirty ways to say I love you. It is the gift that keeps on giving.

Love & Be Loved

Journal Page

Healthy Habits

- Healthy boundaries
- Positive communication
- Self-awareness
- Self-care
- Self-love
- Health & Wellness

A handful of the healthy habits you are cultivating during this process of learning thirty ways to say I love you.

If you come across a term you do not understand, please look it up, and gain a clear understanding of what you are applying to your life.

If you prefer, follow me on any of my social media platforms (Love_light91), direct message me, and we can learn and grow together.

Acknowledgments

To my star seed, Julianne, thank you for the motivation you give me each time I look into your honey brown eyes.

To my ascended angels, Nanny & Aunt Fran, thank you for your wisdom and guidance.

To my grandparents, Robert and Julia —This all started with an egg and glass of water lol.

To my mom, LaSandra —Thank you for being the best friend I never knew I needed.

To my dad, Tony —Thank you for never allowing me to settle, and for pushing me to learn for myself.

To my siblings, Patrick, Nachelle, and TJ—I love you all to through the multiverse and back.

To my editor/publisher— We are Limitless!

Notes

Notes

Notes

Notes

Notes

www.ingramcontent.com/pod-product-compliance
Lightning Source LLC
Chambersburg PA
CBHW071412040426
42444CB00009B/2212